Facial Yoga Secrets: Enhancing Beauty and Relaxation

by

SIRENY FORD

Table of Contents

Summary

If you were told that with 5 simple Face Yoga exercises every day you could tone your facial muscles and prevent them from relaxing, could you spend 3 minutes getting started? Similarly as in recent years we pay great attention to tumbling, fitness and in general to the exercise of our body, so we should likewise pay attention to the fitness of our face. Because that is what Face Yoga is, it's the exercise of the facial muscles!

As strange as it sounds, similarly as we train the muscles of the body, we should prepare the muscles of the face. We might attempt with eye, day, night creams, serums, oils and much more to tighten the skin and not let it relax, however the skincare routine isn't enough by itself and it certainly costs money.

What is face yoga?

Face yoga or face yoga is a program of activities that reinforce facial muscles, restore skin cells and initiate neurons all through the head by arousing region of the facial organs that are not effectively worked out. Fundamentally, it is a mix of tension and back rub in the face and neck region that upgrade blood microcirculation, reestablishing brilliance and imperativeness to pushed skin.

What are the advantages of face yoga?

The advantages of Yoga on the face are above all else mental. The wonderful inclination you have after each face yoga class is reflected in your appearance, the shade of your skin, the radiance of your eyes and the energy you emanate. Simultaneously, the perfusion of the cells and the initiation of the facial muscles make a characteristic guard against the progression of time. In a couple of words, the delicate extending and blood dissemination of the skin coming about because of face yoga, most certainly give your face a more gorgeous appearance.

How It Works

You can consider face yoga a delicate type of "solidarity preparing" for you face and neck muscles. The more you rehash specific face yoga practices that target various pieces of your face, the more you might see that the muscles and skin start to improve somewhat.

In light of what we are familiar facial practices by and large, the face yoga technique appears to work in these ways:

Invigorates facial muscles, working on their tone and "snugness." This can make sense of why it might assist certain individuals with encountering decreased indications of maturing, for example, listing.

Increments blood stream/flow to the skin, which can be useful for clearing skin.

Diminishes strain and pressure in the face muscles that are brought about by rehashed looks over the course of the day, for example, squinting. Back rub and pressure point massage strategies are additionally integrated into the face yoga

technique, loosening up central issues in the face
that will generally become tense.

The Science Behind Face Yoga and Skin Restoration

Embrace an Energetic Gleam with Face Yoga 5 Fundamental Postures

Face yoga has filled in prominence as a characteristic, harmless strategy for skin revival. Despite the fact that there isn't a lot of logical proof with regards to this issue, a few investigations have discovered that a few facial activities might assist with further developing skin quality and muscle tone. The muscles in the face can be reinforced and conditioned with the assistance of facial activities, giving the face a more lifted and young appearance. Moreover, standard facial activities might assist with further developing complexion and surface by supporting blood stream and flow to the face. The completion of their cheeks improved, and the presence of the nasolabial overlay lines that run from the nose to the edges of the mouth was lessened, as per a review that was distributed in the Diary of the American Clinical Affiliation, Dermatology. Members in the review participated in facial activities for quite a long time.

Animating Collagen Creation

The flexibility and solidness of the skin rely upon the protein collagen. Collagen creation declines as we age, bringing about wrinkles, barely recognizable differences, and listing skin. There are, notwithstanding, multiple ways of animating collagen creation and work on your skin's general wellbeing and appearance.

1. Diet: Consuming an eating routine high in cell reinforcements, amino acids, and L-ascorbic acid can uphold the development of collagen. Citrus organic products, salad greens, nuts, and seeds are a couple of food varieties that can assist with keeping up with solid collagen levels.

2. Sun security: UV beams from the sun can hurt collagen filaments, making the skin age rashly. The soundness of your skin can be saved and collagen breakdown can be abstained from by wearing defensive apparel and sunscreen.

3. Skin medicines: Retinoids, peptides, and L-ascorbic acid based skincare items can assist with advancing collagen creation and diminish the presence of scarce differences and kinks.

4. Microneedling: This negligibly obtrusive technique includes utilizing a device with little needles to make minute cuts in the skin, invigorating collagen creation and advancing skin revival.

5. Laser medicines: Some laser methodology, as fragmentary laser reemerging, can work on the surface and tone of the skin and invigorate the development of collagen.

Further developing Blood Course

Great blood course is fundamental for solid skin since it conveys oxygen and supplements to the cells and helps in the expulsion of byproducts. Here are a few ideas for further developing blood course and skin wellbeing:

1. Work out: Ordinary activity increments pulse and enlarges veins, which further develops blood dissemination. No less than 30 minutes of moderate activity, like lively strolling, running, or cycling, ought to be finished every day.

2. Rub: Kneading the skin can energize lymphatic seepage and assist with invigorating blood stream. If you have any desire to further develop dissemination all around, take a stab at utilizing a facial roller or gua sha instrument to rub your face tenderly. You can likewise give yourself a hand or foot rub.

3. Heat treatment: Utilizing intensity to treat the skin can assist with blooding vessels extend and flow get to the next level. Take a stab at utilizing a sauna, a hot shower, or a warm pack on your skin.

4. Hydration: Drying out can make veins contract, so remaining hydrated is basic for keeping up with solid blood stream. Intend to drink no less than 8 cups of water each day.

5. Abstain from smoking: Smoking can limit veins, which diminishes flow and makes the skin age rashly. Quitting any pretense of smoking can improve skin wellbeing and advance general prosperity.

Conditioning Facial Muscles

Conditioning the facial muscles can work on the shape and presence of the face. The accompanying guidance will assist you with conditioning your facial muscles:

1. Practices for the face: Facial activities can help tone and reinforce the face's muscles. Lip handbags, grins, and cheek puffs are a couple of normal facial activities.

2. Facial back rub: A light facial back rub can assist with conditioning the muscles in the face and invigorate blood stream. To rub the skin, have a go at utilizing a gua sha or facial roller.

3. Facial yoga: Facial yoga is like standard yoga in that it includes holding and delivering specific looks to tone and reinforce the muscles in the face.

4. Electrical muscle feeling: By applying gentle electrical flows to the skin, electrical muscle excitement gadgets can assist with conditioning facial muscles.

5. Needle therapy: Needle therapy utilizes minuscule needles embedded into explicit focuses on the face to increment blood stream and fix facial muscles.

Which types of yoga may be better for your face?

Noticing the advantages of yoga asana, customary approaches to sitting during yoga, Specialists makes sense of: "Forward folds carry new blood and oxygen to the skin, which advances a sound gleam. Backbending presents tone and firm the front neck muscles, while turns firm the side of the face and delivery neck strain."

More slow sorts of yoga that include holding models for broadened periods might offer you a greater amount of a chance to carry this attention to your facial muscles. This incorporates Hatha, Yin, or supportive yoga. You can likewise deal with loosening up your face muscles during your intercession, pranayama, or yoga nidra practice.

Work on carrying attention to your face during conventional yoga stances. Notice assuming you're clutching any pressure or making looks. Notice assuming you're focusing on loosening up your face so eagerly that you wind up frowning or lifting your eyebrows.

Which specific areas can doing face yoga exercises help?

Contingent upon your interests and objectives, Specialists says you can utilize face yoga to focus on any region of your face. Pressure will in general form in your temple, foreheads, and jaw. On the off chance that you have snugness in any of these region, assemble your daily schedule around these spots. Wrinkles are normal around the brow, eyes, and mouth.

To lessen the presence of kinks in specific regions, pick back rubs and activities that focus on these spots. Or then again you can pick practices intended to ease explicit worries like migraine, sleep deprivation, or sinus disease.

Which yoga is for beauty?

5 simple yoga asanas for shining skin | Be Lovely India

Sarvangasana (Shoulder Stand Posture)

This posture assists with working on the surface and nature of your skin by elevating blood dissemination to your face thus restoring the platelets. It likewise disposes of skin break out, wrinkles, scarce differences and bluntness.

38 health benefits of yoga

Searching because of motivations to attempt yoga? From expanded strength and adaptability to heart wellbeing, there are 38 advantages to unfurling our bedding.

On the off chance that you're a devoted specialist, you've likely seen a portion of the advantages of yoga — perhaps you rest better or have less colds or simply feel more loose and quiet. However, expecting you've anytime endeavored to enlighten someone else to yoga concerning the benefits of the preparation, you could have found that explanations like "forms the movement of prana" or "raises the energy up the spine" don't click. , , as though addressing a hard of hearing individual or somebody exceptionally incredulous besides.

Researchers are beginning to document the benefits of yoga

Western science has started to give us some strong proof of how yoga further develops wellbeing, mends agony, and keeps sickness under control. At the point when you comprehend this, you'll be extra inspired to step on your sleeping cushion and likely won't feel so silenced the following time

This experience propelled me to dive profound into every one of the logical examinations I gathered in India and the West to find and make sense of how yoga can both forestall sickness and assist you with recuperating from it. I saw this as:

1. Yoga improves your flexibility

Further developed adaptability is perhaps the earliest and most clear advantages of yoga. In your top of the line you likely will not have the option to contact your toes or do a profound backbend. However, in the event that you drive forward, you will see a steady unwinding of the muscles and in the end places that appeared to be difficult to vanquish will start to become conceivable. You will likewise see that the agonies start to vanish. Also, this is no happenstance. Tight hips can overextend the knee joint because of misalignment of the thigh and tibia. Tight biceps can prompt a level lumbar spine which can cause lower back torment.

Solid muscles have a greater number of advantages than simply looking great. They likewise safeguard us from conditions, for example, joint inflammation and lower back torment and assist with forestalling falls in the old, a typical event at this age. Besides, when you foster backbone through yoga you offset it with flexibility.On the off chance that you're about to the exercise center and lifting loads, you will develop fortitude to the detriment of adaptability, so you really want to adjust that too.

Your head resembles a bowling ball: large, round and weighty. At the point when it's decent on your upstanding spine, it takes considerably less work for your neck and back muscles to help it. Move it a couple creeps forward however and you'll begin to extend those muscles. Hold that 'bowling ball' for 8 or 12 hours per day with that forward slant and there's presumably you'll get worn out. Furthermore, exhaustion may not be your main issue. This unfortunate stance can create issues in the midriff, back, neck and different muscles and joints. As you gradually disintegrate,

Each time you do a yoga practice your joints are opened up to their full scope of movement. This can assist with forestalling degenerative joint pain or reduce idleness by packing and de-pressurizing areas of joint ligament that are not regularly utilized. Articular ligament, a flexible connective tissue that interfaces muscle to bone, resembles a wipe: it gets new supplements just when its liquid is pressed out and another stock can be consumed. Without legitimate upkeep disregarded areas of ligament can ultimately erode bringing to the surface and uncovering bone like worn brake cushions on a vehicle.

27

Spinal plates _ which retain shock among vertebrae and can herniate and pack nerves _ need steady development. This is the main way for them to get their supplements. Having an even asana practice with loads of backbends, forward curves and revolutions will assist with keeping these circles adaptable.

It is proven and factual that weight-bearing activities fortify bones and assist with forestalling osteoporosis. Numerous yoga presents expect you to lift your own weight. Furthermore, others like down canine and up canine assist with fortifying the arms, which are especially defenseless against osteoporotic cracks. Unpublished examination from California State College in Los Angeles reports that yoga practice increments bone thickness in the vertebrae. A yoga practice's capacity to bring down levels of the pressure chemical cortisol can assist with keeping up with bone calcium levels.

Yoga gets your blood streaming, gets it going. Specifically, the unwinding practices you learn in yoga can assist with blooding flow, particularly in your arms and legs. Yoga likewise gives more oxygen to your cells, which work much better thus. The turns move blood to the inside organs and permit recently oxygenated blood to circle all through once the revolution is done. Reversals like headstands, uprights, and shoulderstands support venous blood from the legs and pelvis to stream toward the heart, where it very well may be siphoned to the lungs to be oxygenated. This can help in the event that you have enlarged legs because of heart and kidney issues. Yoga likewise helps the degrees of hemoglobin and red platelets which convey oxygen to the tissues. Furthermore, it diminishes the blood by making platelets less tacky and decreasing the degree of clump advancing proteins in the blood. This can prompt a decrease in coronary failures and strokes, as blood clumps are many times the reason for these "executioners".

At the point when you contract and grow your muscles, move your body organs every which way, and get into a yoga position and afterward emerge from that position, you increment the progression of lymph (lymph is a gooey liquid wealthy in safe cells and white platelets that assist with battling contaminations all through the body). This assists the lymphatic framework with battling contamination, obliterate malignant growth cells and discard the harmful materials of cell capability. Assuming that the body is over-burden with poisons and fat, the lymphatic liquids become thick and lumbering. Indeed, we detox through exercise and yoga.

At the point when the pulse is many times in the oxygen consuming reach, then you decrease the gamble of a coronary failure and can ease sadness. While not all that in yoga is vigorous, doing your training live or having a standard astanga or hatha stream practice can support your pulse on a high-impact scale. In any case, even yoga practices that don't raise your pulse can work on cardiovascular guideline. Research has found that rehearsing yoga brings down pulse, increments perseverance, and can further develop top oxygen take-up during exercise — all signs of worked on vigorous wellness. One investigation discovered that individuals who were instructed just pranayama could do more activity with less oxygen.

On the off chance that you have hypertension you might profit from yoga. Two investigations of individuals with hypertension distributed in the English clinical diary 'The Lancet' looked at the impacts of savasana (profound unwinding in dead body present) in a yoga room and essentially lying on a love seat. Following three months, savasana was related with a drop in systolic (or "huge") circulatory strain of 25 places (the biggest number) and a drop in diastolic (or "little") pulse of 15 places (the most reduced number, and the higher the underlying tension the more prominent the drop).

Yoga brings down cortisol levels. On the off chance that that doesn't sound that significant, note this: ordinarily the adrenal organs emit cortisol because of an intense emergency that occasionally helps the resistant framework. Assuming cortisol levels stay high even after the emergency period, the invulnerable framework can be compromised. Occasional expansions in cortisol assist with long haul memory, yet constantly undeniable levels impede memory and can prompt super durable changes in the cerebrum. Moreover, overabundance cortisol has been connected to intense sorrow, osteoporosis (it pulls calcium and different minerals from the bones and disrupts new bone arrangement), hypertension, and insulin obstruction. In mice, elevated degrees of cortisol lead to what analysts call "food-chasing conduct" (the sort that causes you to eat when you're vexed, furious, or focused). The body takes these additional calories and stores them as paunch fat, adding to weight gain and the gamble of diabetes and respiratory failure.

Could it be said that you are feeling miserable? He sat in the lotus position. Even better, get into a backbend or artist's posture. Despite the fact that it is quite difficult, a review presumed that ordinary yoga practice further develops misery and prompts a critical expansion in serotonin levels and a lessening in monoamine oxidase, a chemical that separates synapses, and cortisol levels. At the College of Wisconsin Richard Davidson, Ph.D., found that the left prefrontal cortex showed expanded movement in the people who thought, a finding that connected with more significant levels of satisfaction and better safe capability. Significantly more noteworthy actuation of the left side was tracked down in committed specialists with long haul practice.

Move more, eat less, this is the assessment of numerous nutritionists. Yoga can assist with both. An ordinary practice gets you going while at the same time consuming calories, while the profound and close to home component of the training will urge you to see and manage your eating regimen and weight issues on a more profound level. Yoga can motivate you to eat all the more intentionally.

Yoga brings down glucose and awful cholesterol and lifts great cholesterol. Yoga has been found to bring down glucose levels in individuals with diabetes in more than one way: by bringing down cortisol and adrenaline levels, empowering weight reduction, and further developing aversion with the impacts of insulin. With low sugar levels you decrease the gamble of diabetic complexities, for example, coronary episode, kidney disappointment and visual impairment.

A significant component of yoga is having the option to zero in on the present, the at this point. Research has found that standard yoga practice further develops coordination, response time, memory, and even level of intelligence scores. Individuals who practice supernatural contemplation can tackle issues, secure and review data better, perhaps in light of the fact that they are less diverted by their viewpoints which might play again and again like a perpetual circle.

Yoga urges you to unwind, quiet your breathing and spotlight on the present time and place, moving the equilibrium from the thoughtful sensory system (survival reaction) to the parasympathetic sensory system. The last option loosens up us and prompts recuperation, bringing down breathing and pulses and circulatory strain and expanding blood stream to the digestion tracts and regenerative organs, which incorporates what Herbert Benson, calls the unwinding reaction.

Normal yoga practice increments suddenness, the capacity to feel what your body is doing and where it is in space, and further develops balance. Individuals with unfortunate stance or useless development designs frequently have an unfortunate feeling of proprioception related with knee and lower back issues. Better equilibrium can mean less falls. For the old this converts into additional freedom and a postpone in the time they should be owned up to a medical clinic, or may not be conceded by any means. Until the end of us positions like the tree might cause us to feel less unbalanced all through our bedding.

A few high level yogis have some control over their bodies in a mind blowing manner through their sensory system. Researchers have seen yogis who can inexact extremely uncommon pulses, make unmistakable cerebrum wave examples, and utilizing a contemplation method lift the temperature of their hands by 15 degrees Fahrenheit. On the off chance that they can do this with yoga, we can gain from it to further develop blood stream to the pelvis to get pregnant or to unwind assuming you experience difficulty resting.

Have you at any point saw yourself gripping your telephone or directing wheel or squinting your face while taking a gander at a PC screen? These oblivious propensities can prompt persistent pressure, muscle weakness, and agony in the wrists, arms, shoulders, neck, and face, bringing about expanded tension and low temperament. As you practice yoga you start to see where you gather pressure: it very well might be in the tongue, the eyes or the muscles of the face and neck. Assuming you truly tune in, you might have the option to deliver some strain in the tongue and eyes. For bigger muscles like the quadriceps, trapezius and glutes, it can require long periods of training to figure out how to loosen up them.

Excitement is great, yet in abundance it bothers the sensory system. Yoga can give help from the hurrying around of present day life. Supportive stances, yoga nidra (a type of directed unwinding), the profound unwinding of savasana, pranayama and reflection empower pratyahara, the assimilation of the faculties, which offers time to quiet our sensory system. Another exploration detailed advantage of standard yoga practice is better rest, and that implies you'll be less drained and focused and less inclined to mishaps.

Asanas and pranayama presumably work on safe capability however up to this point reflection has the most grounded logical help around here. It seems to meaningfully affect the capability of the resistant framework, invigorating it when required (eg, bringing neutralizer steps up in light of an immunization) and calming it when required (eg, lessening an undesirable forceful safe capability in an immune system sickness like psoriasis).

Yogis will generally have less breaths during the day yet longer breaths, which is both quieting and powerful. A recent report distributed in the clinical diary "Lancet" exposed a yogic method known as "full relaxing" in individuals with lung issues because of congestive cardiovascular breakdown. Following one month their typical breathing rate dropped from 13.4 breaths each moment to 7.6 breaths. In the mean time, practice limit expanded fundamentally, as did oxygen immersion in their blood. What's more, yoga has been displayed to further develop different lung boundaries, like maximal breathing limit and exhalation productivity.

Yoga additionally energizes breathing through the nose which channels the air, warms it (cold dry air is bound to set off an asthma assault in delicate individuals) and humidifies it eliminating all the soil that is in an ideal situation remaining in your lungs.

Ulcer, crabby gut disorder, obstruction, these can be additionally exasperated by pressure. Well in the event that you stress less you will experience less. Yoga, similar to some other actual activity, can alleviate clogging _ and hypothetically diminish the gamble of colon disease _ in light of the fact that body development works with the fast development of food and waste through the digestion tracts. Also, despite the fact that it has not been logically explored, yogis suspect that turns are gainful exactly in this end of "trash" from our creature.

Yoga stops the variances of the psyche, as indicated by Patanjali's Yoga Sutras . As such, it dials back the psychological circles of bothering, bitterness, outrage, dread and want that cause pressure. Furthermore, since stress is connected to so many medical conditions _ from headaches and a sleeping disorder to lupus, different sclerosis, dermatitis, hypertension and respiratory failure _, in the event that you figure out how to quiet your psyche you'll have a superior opportunity to live longer and better.

A large number of us experience the ill effects of persistent low confidence. Assuming you handle this adversely _ drugs, gorging, difficult work, rest _, you might address the cost of chronic weakness genuinely, intellectually and inwardly. Assuming that you start to adopt a more good strategy and practice yoga, you will feel, at first in a word witnesses yet over the long haul on a more steady premise, that you are commendable or, as yogic way of thinking educates, that you are a sign of the Heavenly. In the event that you have an ordinary practice with the aim of self-investigation, discretion and consistent improvement _ not just as a substitute for a high impact exercise class _, you can move toward an alternate side of yourself. You will encounter sensations of appreciation, compassion and pardoning, as well as a feeling of being a piece of the master plan.

Yoga can ease your aggravation. As per a few examinations, asanas, contemplation, or a blend of both lessens torment in individuals with joint pain, low back torment, fibromyalgia, carpal passage condition, and other ongoing issues. At the point when you assuage your aggravation, your state of mind improves, you choose to be more dynamic and you want less and less drug.

Yoga can assist you with making changes in your day to day existence. This is all there is to it most prominent strength, its most noteworthy benefit, as a matter of fact. Tapas, the Sanskrit word for heat, is the fire, the discipline that powers yoga practice, and that ordinary practice starts to assemble. Tapas, the fire you create, can reach out into numerous aspects of your life to conquer latency and improve on useless propensities. You might find that without putting forth any extraordinary attempt to change things, you will begin eating better, practice more, or at long last stopped smoking following quite a while of bombed endeavors.

Great yoga educators can do ponders for your wellbeing. The excellent ones do significantly more than direct you to a succession of positions. They can address your situation, check when you really want to go further into a position or when you want to return further, let you know hard bits of insight with empathy, assist you with unwinding, and refine and adjust the training to you. A deferential relationship with an educator goes far toward advancing your wellbeing.

In the event that your home medical aid unit helps you to remember a drug store, it very well may be an ideal opportunity to attempt yoga. Investigations of individuals with asthma, hypertension, type II diabetes (supposed grown-up beginning diabetes) and fanatical habitual issue have shown that yoga has assisted them with lessening their prescription dose and at times get off of it out and out. The advantage of taking less medication? You'll spend less cash and be more averse to experience secondary effects and hazard risky medication connections.

Yoga and reflection carry you nearer to mindfulness, increment your degree of mindfulness. Also, the more mindful you are, the simpler it is to dispose of damaging feelings like resentment. Research shows that constant indignation and aggression are as firmly connected to cardiovascular failure as smoking, diabetes and elevated cholesterol levels. Yoga seems to decrease outrage by expanding sensations of sympathy and connectedness and loosening up the sensory system and brain. It additionally builds the capacity to move away from the show of your life and stay immovable notwithstanding terrible news or disturbing occasions.

Love may not overcome all, however it sure mends. Developing daily reassurance from companions, family and local area has been over and over displayed to further develop wellbeing and mending. A standard yoga practice assists you with creating benevolence, sympathy and more prominent harmony. Alongside yogic way of thinking's accentuation on abstaining from hurting others, coming clean, and having just what we want, this can work on large numbers of our connections.

The underpinnings of yoga — asana, pranayama and reflection — assist with working on your wellbeing, yet there's something else entirely to the yoga tool stash, such as singing. It broadens your exhalation, which moves the equilibrium towards the parasympathetic sensory system. At the point when done in a gathering, singing can be an especially strong physical and profound experience. A new report from the Karolinska Foundation in Sweden shows that murmuring sounds like the one we make while reciting Om open the sinuses and work with waste.

In the event that you suppose, assuming you structure a picture to you as you do for example in yoga nidra and different practices, you can influence change in your body. Some exploration has found that directed representation decreased postoperative torment, diminished the recurrence of migraines, and worked on personal satisfaction in individuals with disease and HIV.

Kriyas or purifying and detoxification strategies are one more component of yoga. They incorporate all that from speedy breathing activities to inward entrail purging. Jala neti, which is a delicate washing of the nasal sections with salt water, eliminates pollutants and infections from the nose, forestalls bodily fluid development and helps channel the sinuses.

Karma yoga (administration to other people) is a basic piece of yogic way of thinking. And keeping in mind that you may not be leaned to help other people, your wellbeing can be significantly improved assuming you do. A College of Michigan investigation discovered that more established individuals who chipped in less than an hour seven days were multiple times bound to be alive a couple of years after the fact. Serving and helping other people can give your life meaning and your concerns may not appear to be so alarming when you see what others are carrying on with in their lives.

In a ton of customary medicine most patients are disconnected recipients of care. In yoga how counts is what you help yourself. Yoga gives you the instruments to change and you'll begin feeling better whenever you first practice. You will likewise see that the more predictable you are in your training the more prominent the advantages. This is a direct result of three things: you engaged in taking care of oneself, you found that your contribution empowered you to influence change, and by seeing the change you started to trust. Also, trust itself can mend.

As you read through every one of the manners in which yoga further develops wellbeing, you might see a ton of cross-over. This is on the grounds that they are firmly interwoven. Change your stance and the manner in which you inhale will change. Change your breathing and you will change your sensory system. This is perhaps of the best illustration in yoga. Everything is associated _ hip to lower leg, you and your local area, your local area to the world. This association is essential to grasping yoga. This all encompassing framework all the while includes numerous instruments that make added substance and multiplicative impacts. This cooperative energy is maybe the main method of all that yoga recuperates.

Also, simply accepting that you will get well can make you well. Sadly numerous traditional medication researchers trust that on the off chance that something works utilizing a fake treatment it doesn't count. Be that as it may, numerous patients simply need to recover, so if reciting a mantra, as finished toward the start and end of a yoga practice or during a contemplation or day, works with recuperating, regardless of whether it is a self-influenced consequence, why not don't make it happen?

What is the best time to do yoga?

There is no particular season of day when yoga practice ought to be stayed away from, for however long it isn't after a feast. While rehearsing yoga in the first part of the day can make numerous positive impacts, there are motivations to rehearse in the early evening or night, separately, and ways of upgrading your experience in view of when you practice yoga. Picking the best chance to do yoga is totally private.

Morning yoga practice

Rehearsing yoga in the first part of the day is an extraordinary method for extending your body and set it up until the end of the day. Yoga invigorates blood dissemination and numerous organ capabilities, which is an incredible method for beginning the morning before an energy sapping workday. Additionally, clearing and calming the brain and thinking in the first part of the day, with profound full breaths and breath control works out (pranayama), will assist with diminishing feelings of anxiety and increment your concentration, fixation. Likewise, rehearsing yoga not long before day break is a customary strategy that is viewed as the best time for otherworldly practice (sadhana).

Afternoon yoga practice

Assuming you feel that your muscles are extremely firm in the first part of the day, rehearsing yoga can be truly pleasant and assist you with extending your muscles better. Nonetheless, on the off chance that morning practice isn't for you, holding on until some other time in the day will permit you substantially more opportunity of development as your body will have heated up during the day. Being more agreeable in your developments will loosen up you making it simpler for you to clear your psyche and assuage pressure that has developed during the day. Additionally, assuming you feel that yoga assists with your assimilation, rehearsing later in the day can assist you with managing the a throbbing painfulness you hope to feel around evening time or in the first part of the day.

Rehearsing yoga at night can unbelievably unwind. On the off chance that you feel snugness in your back and experience difficulty dozing around evening time, certain asanas can truly assist with easing pressure in your lower back and legs for a more tranquil rest. There are even places that are protected and agreeable to perform while in bed. Rehearsing yoga at night can cause you to feel more great in the event that you experience morning affliction or uneasiness.

Regardless of what the best time is for you, it is sure that a yoga practice will bring positive outcomes and different advantages.

Other factors

At last, one more element to consider is the climate. In winter early morning yoga practice can make your muscles and lungs self-conscious on the off chance that the air is dry. Summer can be too blistering to even consider rehearsing around mid-afternoon, so you might need to move your training to the morning or night after dusk. The key is to be agreeable, generally your consideration and center will disappear during the training and you might start to feel troubled as opposed to loose.

Face Yoga Exercises

In contrast to certain sorts of yoga, for example, Bikram or Ashtanga, there isn't one standard face yoga grouping to adhere to. Maybe there are heaps of various activities you can attempt, in no specific request, to check whether they give you any advantages or help.

In one review, 32 particular facial activities were polished, every one for about a moment. Cases of various exercises integrated those zeroing in on the lower and upper cheek, space around the eyes, facial design, neck and mid temple.

The exercises were suggested by names, for example,

- Cheek lifter
- Eyebrow lifter
- Cheerful cheeks chiseling
- Scooping: jaw and neck firmer
- Sanctuary designer
- Upper eyelid firmer

Coming up next are assortments of some notable face yoga rehearses you can practice at home:

[*Note: Make an effort not to wrinkle your face excessively or squint while playing out these activities, which can be counterproductive. Focal point of lifting and growing instead.]

1. Stunner

Utilize your fingers to frame "binocular" shape around your eyebrows, cheeks and across the face. Lift your eyebrows without wrinkling the temple to an extreme, then squint and afterward lift them once more. Intend to rehash multiple times.

2. Brow Lifter

Interweave your fingers over your brow and apply light tension while endeavoring to lift your temple. Rehash multiple times, as well as hold for as long as one moment.

One more method for doing this is to put the two palms on your sanctuaries, push your palms up and back to lift the sides of your face, then hold for five seconds and continue to rehash.

3. Cheek Lifter

Open your mouth wide, keep your tooth masking your lips and raise your cheeks. Hold for 10 seconds, then get back to business as usual. Mean to rehash multiple times. (Do whatever it takes not to squint while lifting.)

4. Neck and Jaw Stretch

Incline your face up fairly, then, at that point, lift your jaw up and progress at a 45-degree point and over toward one shoulder, holding there for three seconds.Get once again to focus, then, at that point, rehash to the opposite side. Rehash multiple times on each side, or expect to continue to rehash for one or a few minutes in a row.

One more effective method for extending and reinforcing your neck and jaw (provided that you have no neck issues) is to shift your head as far as possible back and hold, rehashing for as long as a moment.

5. Pucker Lips

Pucker your lips, release them somewhat and rehash. Rehash for dependent upon one or a few minutes.

6. Smiler

Grin more than one times without wrinkling your eyes, then, at that point, keep a delicate grin for fifty seconds in a row.

7. Knead + Face Savasana

Clean your hands and face with a delicate cleaning agent, then rub your face everywhere (you might need to utilize coconut oil to make this simpler). Tenderly press your fingertips into your facial muscles to assuage any strain. Make a point to focus on your "third eye" (the space between your temples), kneading for 30 minutes and circumnavigating around your eyes. (You might need to have a go at utilizing your fits around your brow and eyes as well.)

Get done with a warm towel laid over your face as you set down and unwind.

6 yoga poses that can give you bright and glowing skin

Yoga is known to give you an adaptable and fit body, however have you considered doing yoga for skin health management? Check it out.

These are not many asanas of yoga for healthy skin:

1. Bow Pose (Dhanurasana)

This posture of yoga for healthy skin works successfully in giving you a gleaming composition. Rehearsing this posture routinely helps by coming down on the stomach district, which thusly helps in detoxifying the body. This posture increments course in the face and pelvic locale. It lets pressure out of the midsection and fortifies it. Standard act of this asana reinforces the regenerative organs. It likewise helps discharge acid reflux and clogging. By keeping a sound stomach, dhanurasana helps in giving you that shining and solid skin appearance.

How to do this yoga asana

- Rests on the floor level on your stomach. Twist your legs from the knee keeping your knee hip-width separated. Broaden your hands behind and snatch your lower legs from an external perspective.

- Breathe in, and light your entire body off the floor adjusting on the navel

- Breathe out, and gradually discharge the position.

2. Seated Forward Bend (Paschimottanasana)

This is a wonderful asana to extend the spine, shoulders and hamstrings. It delivers the pressure in the lower back and furthermore further develops absorption, which in any case might cause many skin conditions like pimples and skin inflammation. Not exclusively is this posture useful for diminishing pressure, it additionally decontaminates the blood, further develops skin coloring and lessens the presence of dull spots and kinks. Paschimottasana is an ideal yoga for skin health management.

How to do this yoga asana

- Begin by sitting on the floor with your legs broadened straight ahead.
- Place your feet together and flex your feet towards you. Breathe in, fix the spine upwards.
- Breathe out, lean your chest area forward, bowing from the hip, keeping a straight spine while twisting forward.

3. Downward-facing dog (Adho Mukha Svanasana)

According to shetty, "This asana loosens up the whole body. It fortifies the arms and shoulders, extends the spine, calves and hamstrings and stimulates the whole body by bringing blood stream to your mind and face." This asana further develops blood course in those areas giving you solid flushed cheeks.

How to do this yoga asana

- Begin the floor by setting your hands and knees down.
- Fix your legs by taking your knees off the floor and push your heels down to the extent that they can go. Expand the spine by driving away starting from the earliest stage your palms.
- Remain in the posture for 5 to 9 breaths.

4. Fish Pose (Matsyasana)

Fish present is one of the back-bowing represents that can be effortlessly performed even by a novice. This is one of the most amazing yoga postures to accomplish new and, surprisingly, conditioned skin as it further develops blood dissemination in the head district.

How to do this yoga asana

- Sit in a Padmasana yoga present.
- Gradually twist in reverse and put your head on the ground.
- As you contact the ground with the highest point of your head, lift your chest upwards.
- Hold the stance for several minutes.

5. Plough Pose (Halasana)

This yoga present is successful in further developing the general blood flow of the body. It prompts a vibe of serenity and places you in a casual perspective making it an ideal posture of yoga for skin health management.

"This posture is advantageous in prompting rest or handling sleep deprivation considering the way that unfortunate rest cycle is one of the significant explanations for awful skin conditions. This multitude of constructive outcomes of this asana think about your skin," .

How to do this yoga asana

- Rests on your back, palms confronting the roof.
- Delicately lift your legs at ninety degrees and take them over your head to contact the flour.
- Keep up with the posture briefly, return to ordinary position

6. Shoulder stand (Sarvangasana)

This would be a halfway level posture which has astonishing advantages on your skin and sparkle. Dominating this posture is actually somewhat straightforward, ordinary practice helps in further developing blood dissemination to the facial area, which assists in engaging with cleaning conditions like facial bluntness, skin break out and wrinkles.

How to do this yoga asana

- Set down on your back, confronting the roof.
- Tenderly lift your legs and hips straight up by supporting back with your hands.
- Stay in the situation for a couple of moments; return to the typical position.

Safety measures to Take With Face Yoga

A few specialists say that facial yoga might make wrinkles due the dull developments of the skin. At the point when you more than once contract your facial muscles, this could really make wrinkles structure. As you age, your skin normally loses collagen and elastin. A lot rubbing or control of your skin might expand its deficiency of flexibility.

Rehashed compression of specific pieces of your upper face, like your brow, crow's feet, and grimace lines can make those lines further over the long haul.

Specialists say that face yoga's enemy of maturing impacts might require three to about a month prior to results should be visible. You likewise must be predictable with facial yoga practices 6 days to 7 days per week. Do the activities for 20 minutes to 30 minutes every day.

Converse with your PCP prior to beginning facial yoga. Face yoga may not be for everybody. In the event that you've had restorative injectables like dermal fillers, face yoga might make the fillers keep going for a more limited time frame.

How to Reduce Premature Skin Aging

Here are another ways of diminishing untimely skin maturing:

Use sun security. Apply sunscreen consistently to all the skin that is not covered by apparel. Use sunscreen that is water-safe, wide range, and SPF 30 or higher. Safeguard your skin by wearing sun-defensive apparel and remaining in the shade whenever the situation allows.

1. Quit smoking. Smoking causes wrinkles and a dull coloring. It likewise ages your skin all the more rapidly.
2. Drink less liquor. Liquor can cause dry skin and, over the long run, causes skin harm.
3. Eat an even eating regimen. An eating regimen high in sugar and refined carbs can accelerate maturing.
4. Eat new vegetables and organic products to help sound skin.

5. Abstain from tanning, whether from a tanning bed or from the sun. The UV light from tanning rashly ages your skin.

6. Work-out consistently. Practice helps support your safe framework and works on your course.

7. Clean up two times every day and after you sweat a ton. Sweat bothers your skin, particularly while you're wearing a head protector or cap.

8. Saturate everyday. Lotion keeps your skin hydrated, making it look more energetic.

Embrace an Energetic Sparkle with Face Yoga: 5 Fundamental Stances

Face yoga, otherwise called facial yoga or facial activities, is a characteristic method for working on the wellbeing and presence of your skin and accomplish an energetic sparkle. The following are five fundamental face yoga represents that will assist you with looking more energetic and brilliant:

- The muscles around the cheeks and mouth are lifted and conditioned by this posture. Put your list and center fingers on each hand looking like a V and put them on the sides of your mouth to pause dramatically. Indent your skin with your fingers while smiling extensively. Hold for 10 seconds, unwind, and rehash.

- This position focuses on the muscles around the eyes, which further develops complexion and lessens wrinkles. Beginning with the external corners of your eyes, delicately pull the skin there toward your sanctuaries utilizing your pointers. While standing firm on this situation, lift your eyebrows all over. Rehash multiple times.

- This position helps with limiting kinks and scarce differences around the mouth and jawline. Begin by puckering your lips and sucking your cheeks in. Hold for 5 seconds, then, at that point, discharge. Rehash multiple times.

- The neck muscles are the focal point of this posture, which additionally further develops complexion and diminishes drooping. Begin by putting your fingertips on your collarbone and looking up at the roof. While keeping your head here, slant your head back and present your jaw. Hold for 10 seconds, then, at that point, discharge. Rehash multiple times.

- This position focuses on the muscles in the mouth locale and attempts to limit grin lines. Begin by gently pushing down with your pointers on the edges of your mouth. Grin as wide as possible while keeping your fingers set up. Hold for 10 seconds, then, at that point, discharge. Rehash multiple times.

The Forehead Smoother: Reducing Forehead Lines

Temple lines are a typical indication of maturing, however there are multiple ways of diminishing their appearance. Here are a few ways to accomplish a smoother, more energetic looking brow:

1. Customary facial activities can assist the muscles in the temple with becoming more grounded and more conditioned, which can assist with diminishing the perceivability of lines and kinks. Have a go at performing practices like raising and bringing down your temples or squeezing back against your fingertips with your fingertips on your brow.

2. Delicately kneading your face can assist with expanding blood stream, empower the development of collagen in your skin, and reduce the presence of lines and kinks.

Attempt delicately kneading the brow in round movements utilizing your fingertips.

3. It very well may be gainful to keep the skin on your brow saturated to reduce the presence of lines and kinks. Use a lotion with hostile to maturing parts like retinol or hyaluronic corrosive to assist the skin with turning out to be more flexible and to support the development of collagen.

4. By safeguarding your skin from the sun's harming UV beams, you can stop further crumbling and decrease the perceivability of lines and kinks. Break a cap or look for down cover from the sun when you can, and utilize expansive range sunscreen with basically SPF 30.

5. Botox, a typical restorative method, briefly incapacitates the muscles that cause kinks and temple lines, assisting with lessening

their appearance. Looking for proficient exhortation prior to pursuing this choice is vital.

The Cheek Lifter: Conditioning Cheek Muscles

Conditioning the cheek muscles can assist lift and firm the cheeks, which with canning work on the general appearance of the face. Here are a few ways to condition the cheek muscles:

1. There are a few facial activities that can assist with conditioning the cheek muscles, incorporating grinning with your mouth shut, sucking your cheeks in, and blowing air into your cheeks like an inflatable. Rehash these activities a few times each day to help tone and lift the cheek muscles.

2. Face yoga includes utilizing yoga postures and breathing strategies to tone and lifts the facial muscles. Some face yoga represents that can assist with conditioning the cheek muscles incorporate the cheek lift, the fish face, and the grinning fish face.

3. Delicately kneading the cheeks can assist with further developing blood stream and animate collagen creation, which can help tone and lift the cheek muscles. Take a stab at utilizing up strokes with your fingertips to knead the cheeks tenderly.

4. Facial rollers, which are regularly made of jade or different gemstones, can assist with invigorating blood stream and advance lymphatic waste, which can assist with lessening puffiness and tone the cheek muscles. Utilize the roller to rub the cheeks in a vertical movement tenderly.

5. Drinking a lot of water and eating a reasonable eating regimen that is plentiful in nutrients and cell reinforcements can assist with supporting solid skin and muscle capability. This can assist with working on the tone and lift of the cheek muscles over the long haul.

The Angular shape: Firming Facial structure and Neck

Accomplishing an Angular face with a firm facial structure and neck can cause your face to show up more young and characterized. Here are a few ways to firm your facial structure and neck:

1. Normal facial activities can help diminish hanging and upgrade the general appearance of the face by reinforcing and conditioning the muscles in the facial structure and neck. Take a stab at performing practices like jaw grasps, neck stretches, and jaw lifts.

2. Face yoga can support lifting and conditioning facial muscles, remembering those for the neck and facial structure. The jaw fold, tongue stretch, and neck roll are a couple of face yoga represents that can help tone the facial structure and neck.

3. Retinol, L-ascorbic acid, and hyaluronic corrosive are instances of fixings found in

skincare items that can assist with further developing skin flexibility and solidness, which can assist with diminishing hanging in the neck and facial structure.

4. Unfortunate stance can add to hanging in the facial structure and neck. Keeping up with appropriate stance, for example, sitting upright and keeping your jaw lined up with the floor, can help your facial structure and neck look better.

5. Practices planned explicitly for the neck muscles can help tone and reinforce the region notwithstanding facial activities. The facial structure and neck can be more appealing with practices like head slants, neck stretches, and opposition band exercises.

The Eye Brightener: Lifting Eyebrows and Decreasing Crow's Feet

The eye region is a typical area of worry for some individuals with regards to indications of maturing. Here are a few suggestions for temple lifting works out, face yoga, eye creams, botox, shades, and sunscreen to give you a more energetic, excited appearance. You can assist with lifting your eyebrows and diminish the presence of crow's feet for a more energetic, excited appearance by integrating these tips into your skincare and work-out daily practice. Remember that it could require some investment before you get results, so be patient, and assuming you have any worries, converse with an expert.

The Lip Plumper: Smoothing and Upgrading Lips

Your appearance can be improved and you can seem more youthful by having lips that are smooth, full, and stout. Here are a few hints for smoothing and upgrading your lips:

1. Shedding: Eliminating dead skin cells and advancing cell turnover through standard peeling of your lips can assist with relaxing and smoothen them. Have a go at utilizing a lip scour or tenderly brushing your lips with a delicate shuddered toothbrush.

2. Hydration: Keeping up with hydrated lips is fundamental for getting smooth, stout lips. Utilize a lip medicine or oil to assist with securing in dampness and hydrate.

3. Facial activities: Normal facial activities can further develop blood flow and tone the muscles around the lips, improving their

shape and completion. Explore different avenues regarding activities, for example, the lip press and the grin smoother.

4. Lip-plumping items: By supporting blood stream and giving your lips a short plumping impact, lip-plumping items like lip medicine, serums, and shines can assist with working on their appearance. Search for items that incorporate peptides and hyaluronic corrosive among their fixings.

5. Lip fillers: Lip fillers can assist with adding volume and smooth out scarcely discernible differences and kinks for a more extended enduring lip improvement. Just a prepared and authorized proficient ought to carry out this operation.

Ways to integrate Face Yoga into Your Daily practice

Embrace an Energetic Sparkle with Face Yoga: 5 Fundamental Stances

Here are a few ideas to kick you off on the off chance that you're keen on adding face yoga to your everyday practice:

1. Begin with a warm-up: To keep away from injury, it's essential to heat up your facial muscles before beginning your face yoga practice. Have a go at heating up your hands by scouring them together, then put your palms all over and give your skin a light back rub.

2. Find a serene, agreeable region: Since rehearsing face yoga requires concentration and focus, it's basic to find a tranquil, agreeable region where you can do as such without interference.

3. Follow an everyday practice: While performing face yoga, it very well may be gainful to adhere to a bunch of postures or a daily schedule. You can do this to keep up with your fixation and ensure you're focusing on every one of the fundamental facial regions.

4. Practice routinely: Consistency is key with regards to confront yoga. To begin getting results, attempt to rehearse basically a couple of times each week.

5. Show restraint: It could require an investment for face yoga to begin working, so being patient and proceed with your practice is significant. Maintain at the top of the priority list that face yoga enjoys benefits past working on your skin's appearance; it can likewise assist you with adapting to pressure and feel better all over.

6. Join face yoga with other skincare schedules: Dealing with your skin from an external perspective in is similarly just about as significant as involving face yoga as a feature of your general skincare routine. Make certain to purge, saturate, and safeguard your skin with sunscreen to assist with keeping an energetic coloring.

Consistency is Key for Apparent Outcomes

Consistency is fundamental for accomplishing apparent outcomes with face yoga or some other taking care of oneself practice. Face yoga, regardless of whether just for a couple of moments daily, can assist with working on the tone, surface, and in general appearance of your skin. Notwithstanding, remember that everybody's skin is unique, and results might shift relying upon factors like age, skin type, and generally wellbeing. Certain individuals might get results after half a month of predictable practice, while others might require additional time. Notwithstanding steady practice, it is basic to be patient and delicate with your skin. Applying a lot of tension or pulling too severe with your skin can cause harm and perhaps demolish the presence of barely recognizable differences and kinks. Face yoga ought to be joined with other solid propensities, for example, remaining hydrated, getting sufficient rest, and eating a fair eating routine. You can uphold the wellbeing and presence of your skin by dealing with your body from the back to front.

Match Face Yoga with a Decent Skincare Routine

You can obtain improved results by consolidating face yoga with an even skincare schedule. Here are a few pointers for fostering an even skincare routine to supplement your face yoga practice.

1. Purify: To begin, peel your skin to dispose of any soil, oil, and debasements. Make a point to utilize a delicate chemical that won't dry out your skin or eliminate its regular oils.

2. Tone: To adjust the pH of your skin and prepare it until the end of your skincare schedule, utilize a toner next. Search for a toner that contains quieting fixings like rosewater or chamomile and is liberated from cruel synthetic substances.

3. Saturate: In the wake of conditioning, apply a cream to help hydrate and safeguard your skin. Find a cream that is reasonable for

your skin type and contains sustaining parts like hyaluronic corrosive or vitamin E.

4. Safeguard: Protecting your skin from the harming impacts of UV radiation during the day is pivotal. Prior to heading outside, utilize expansive range sunscreen with a SPF of something like 30.

5. Treat: Contingent upon your skin's prerequisites, you could likewise need to incorporate particular skincare items like serums or covers in your everyday practice. To assist with decreasing the presence of scarce differences, wrinkles, and different indications of maturing, search for items that contain fixings like retinol, L-ascorbic acid, or peptides.

Join Face Yoga with Other Pressure Help Methods

Stress is a significant supporter of various skin issues, like scarce differences, kinks, and bluntness. You can assist with supporting the wellbeing and presence of your skin from the back to front by consolidating face yoga with other pressure alleviation strategies. Here are some pressure alleviation strategies to consider:

1. Reflection: Contemplation can assist with quieting your brain and decrease feelings of anxiety. Have a go at saving a couple of moments every day to contemplate, either all alone or utilizing a directed reflection application.

2. Yoga: Participating in yoga activities can assist you with feeling more loose and amazing generally speaking. Ponder consolidating hatha or vinyasa yoga into

your everyday practice notwithstanding face yoga.

3. Profound breathing activities: Profound breathing activities can ease pressure and energize unwinding. Put in no time flat consistently taking a couple of slow, full breaths in through your nose and out through your mouth.

4. Fragrant healing: A few aromas, similar to lavender or chamomile, are prestigious for being quieting. Use quieting natural ointments or consume candles to take a stab at integrating fragrant healing into your everyday practice.

5. Care: Care involves being completely participated in the job that needs to be done and zeroing in on the current second. Whether you're doing the dishes, taking a walk, or investing energy with friends and

family, have a go at rehearsing care over the course of the day.

Extra Advantages of Face Yoga Past Skin Wellbeing

Embrace a Young Gleam with Face Yoga: 5 Fundamental Postures

Face yoga, notwithstanding its skin medical advantages, has various different benefits for both the psyche and the body. Following are a few extra benefits to rehearsing face yoga:

1. Stress decrease: Face yoga, as different types of yoga, can support facilitating strain and empowering unwinding. Face yoga utilizes care and profound breathing to assist with quieting the brain and diminish strain and restless sentiments.

2. Further developed facial muscle tone: Face yoga can help bind together and reinforce your facial muscles, which can upgrade the evenness and equilibrium of your face all in all. This might bring about a more lifted, energetic appearance.

3. Expanded course: Face yoga can assist with further developing skin surface and tone by expanding blood stream to the face. A better, more brilliant tone and less puffiness might benefit from some intervention by further developed course.

4. Worked on look: Rehearsing face yoga can show you how to more readily control your looks and become more aware of them. This can make it simpler for you to impart, and it could try and assist with reducing the presence of almost negligible differences and kinks welcomed on by rehashed looks.

5. Worked on relaxing: Profound breathing activities, which are a critical part of face yoga, can assist with bettering lung capability and respiratory wellbeing overall.

Decreasing Pressure and Nervousness

One of the many benefits of face yoga is that it assists with decreasing pressure and nervousness. Notwithstanding the profound breathing and care procedures utilized in face yoga, there are other pressure decrease techniques you can attempt. The following are a couple of ideas:

1. Work out: Customary active work, like yoga, strolling, or swimming, discharges endorphins, the body's normal lighthearted chemicals, which can assist with bringing down pressure and nervousness.

2. Rest: For overseeing pressure and tension, it is critical to get sufficient rest. To assist you with unwinding before bed, lay out a quieting sleep time routine and go for the gold long periods of rest every evening.

3. Care: Utilizing strategies like profound breathing activities or reflection, you can figure out how to be more aware of your environmental elements and keep up with your consideration, which will assist you with feeling less worried and restless.

4. Social help: Making loved ones associations or joining a care group can encourage a feeling of having a place and reduce pressure and sensations of forlornness.

5. Taking care of oneself: Dealing with oneself by doing things like cleaning up, perusing a book, or going outside can assist with easing pressure and support unwinding.

Upgrading Care and Concentration

Face yoga can likewise assist you with working on your care and concentration. You can prepare your psyche to remain present and zeroed in on the main job by rehearsing the activities carefully. Here are a few pointers to assist you with working on your care and concentration during your face yoga practice:

1. Set an aim: Set an aim for what you need to accomplish or zero in on during your face yoga practice before you start. This could go from diminishing temple pressure to expanding breath mindfulness.

2. Center around your breath: One of the main parts of care is focusing on your relaxing. Focus on your breath as you travel through your face yoga practice and attempt to keep it consistent and loose.

3. Remain present: During yoga practice, it's simple for the psyche to meander, so attempt to remain present and zeroed in on the developments and impressions of each activity. On the off chance that your brain meanders, tenderly take it back to your breath and the development of your body.

4. Practice routinely: Consistency is key with regards to improving care and concentration. Attempt to rehearse face yoga simultaneously every day, and hold back nothing length of training to assist with preparing your brain to remain present and centered.

5. Limit interruptions: To improve care and concentration, attempt to limit interruptions during your training. Switch off your telephone, track down a calm space to rehearse, and take out some other likely interruptions.

End: Experience the Age-opposing Force of Face Yoga

Embrace an Energetic Sparkle with Face Yoga: 5 Fundamental Stances

Face yoga is an all encompassing and normal strategy for skin revival that offers many benefits as well as reducing the presence of scarce differences and kinks. By integrating face yoga into your everyday daily practice, you can support the creation of collagen, upgrade blood flow, and tone facial muscles for a composition that looks more energetic. Alongside these actual benefits, face yoga can assist with pressure and tension decrease, care and center upgrade, and general prosperity advancement. Face yoga can help your skin's wellbeing while likewise improving your overall wellbeing and prosperity when joined with an even skincare normal and other pressure easing methods. Recall that consistency is fundamental for seeing noticeable outcomes from face yoga. You can encounter the age-opposing force of face yoga and partake in a more energetic looking coloring into the indefinite future by rehearsing consistently and paying attention to your body's requirements.

End: Experience the Age-opposing Force of Face Yoga

Embrace an Energetic Sparkle with Face Yoga: 5 Fundamental Stances

Face yoga is an all encompassing and normal strategy for skin revival that offers many benefits as well as reducing the presence of scarce differences and kinks. By integrating face yoga into your everyday daily practice, you can support the creation of collagen, upgrade blood flow, and tone facial muscles for a composition that looks more energetic. Alongside these actual benefits, face yoga can assist with pressure and tension decrease, care and center upgrade, and general prosperity advancement. Face yoga can help your skin's wellbeing while likewise improving your overall wellbeing and prosperity when joined with an even skincare normal and other pressure easing methods. Recall that consistency is fundamental for seeing noticeable outcomes from face yoga. You can encounter the age-opposing force of face yoga and partake in a more energetic looking coloring into the indefinite future by rehearsing consistently and paying attention to your body's requirements.